Her Motivational Code

Forget and Leave Self-Doubt, Build self-Confidence, and Embrace Who You Are.

BY

Chrissie Borg
The Fox Books

About the Author

 Chrissie Borg is a professor and life coach with expert knowledge in Behavioral Psychology. She has extensive knowledge from ten years of working in the different fields of human Psychology, with hundreds of couples, women, and parents seeking her advice and using it to flourish in their lives.

She focuses on assisting couples in embracing compassion, connection, and good communication skills, arguing that intimate relationships require effort from both partners to work. She has a deep insight into what causes the couple's disputes and how to resolve them. Throughout her career, she has assisted hundreds of couples in improving their married life by working on their communication and conflict management skills.

She has provided Therapy to many individuals suffering from BPD to help them lead a useful life. Providing counseling and treatment to people suffering from mental disorders, helping couples and parents improve their family relations, time management, building confidence in women, and improving the quality of life through healthy habits are some of her favorite writing topics.

Table of contents

Introduction

According to global research released by The Body Shop, one in every two women feels more self-doubt than self-love, and 60 percent wish they had more respect for themselves.

Now that is a self-love crisis!

Let me paint a picture of my past that might sound familiar to you.

"My friend, who is visiting me, is sprawled on my bed as we go through one of our regular rituals: I rummage through my closet and offer her the items I do not wear anymore. "Take this," I say, "I don't have the legs for short skirts," or "These pants make me appear like a hippy." She looks at me puzzled as if I have body dysmorphic disorder, in which I am fixated with minor and frequently fictional imperfections in my physical appearance. She insists that I need new glasses at the very least."

We are not just talking about bodily insecurity here. When I met with a book editor about a potential publication contract, I was concerned about my talents, despite a successful career and a long-standing reputation. If I had dinner guests, I would worry that my house would not look nice, that my brownies would not be worth the calories, and that the conversation would not be interesting enough.

Still, I managed to get by in life, earning a living and maintaining relationships. However, when I saw the film Pretty Woman, it came to me that many of us suffer from the same self-doubt that wrecked Julia Roberts' character. She tells a wealthy businessman played by Richard Gere that no one ever plans to be a hooker and that she has stumbled into this line of work because she has not thought highly of herself. Gere thinks she is a unique individual with a lot of potential and ability. "The bad stuff is easier to believe," she explains.

Why is it that certain people, like Donald Trump, appear to believe only the greatest things about themselves? In contrast, others, particularly women, seize on the most self-critical thoughts they can have? It turns out that negative thinking is tied to a certain part of your brain. The anterior cingulate cortex is a worrywart area of the brain. It is actually larger and more influential in women, as is the brain circuitry for observing other people's emotions. We believe females have greater emotional sensitivity because we have been designed to respond quickly to the requirements of a nonverbal infant.

Women often undervalue their own abilities. Most male managers think their best female colleagues lack assertiveness. Furthermore, extensive research demonstrates that women will not pursue promotions or new assignments if they believe there is even a small probability of failure. Men are significantly more risk-tolerant, and a lot more likely to believe they will succeed.

Moreover, women are perfectionists. It makes feeling good about ourselves much more difficult. We have a habit of dwelling on our errors. I read great literature alongside great intellectuals, and one of my teachers even suggested that I might have a future in academia. But that is not what I recall most of the time. What comes to mind is a class where I read the word "espresso" wrong. For a lot of years, this memory found me filled with shame.

The difference in how boys and girls were socialized a generation ago was widely blamed for the confidence gap. Girls were brought up to be shyer, with lesser expectations allowing boys to take the lead. It was said that girls' confidence would rise if we encouraged them to play with cars and encouraged teachers to give them due attention in class.

Things are different now. In school, girls outperform their male peers. They are more adept at adhering to regulations and fulfilling commitments. However, when they enter the professional world, the men emerge victoriously. Why?

Evolutionary psychology and modern brain science have largely dismantled the blank-slate notion of gender differences. It is known that female and male brains differ somewhat and that these variations, together with hormones, significantly impact personality and behavior.

Is that it for us? No, our minds are adaptable. We can modify our emotions and actions with practice and persistence. This is my inspiration for writing this book. Knowing your self-worth and believing in it can do wonders to your life.

You are enough. You are capable. You can do everything. You are very much deserving of love and affection.

This book is devoted to motivating women to realize their potential and self-worth and believe in it. The first chapter of the book is focused on breaking free from the trap of self-doubt with effective strategies. The second chapter is all about boosting your self-confidence so you can freely celebrate and be your unique and worthy self in front of the world. The third chapter hovers over self-acceptance and self-love. It emphasizes your right to be loved and deserve everything well.

Who am I to you? What does it matter what I say? I am a life coach with ten years of experience. I meet with women like you every day, struggling to find their self-worth when they are, in fact, brilliant and beautiful. I myself have had years of self-doubt and self-hate, to be honest. This all changed when I had a daughter of my own. Just telling her a few worn-out statements about self-love would not teach her to love, respect, and believe in herself. I needed to show her. I also realized how unfair I was to myself. Safe to say, I cried a lot when I did. It sparked a purpose inside me. I put my job as an English professor behind me and started training as a life coach. I want no one to feel any less about themselves and live a life they are proud of.

This book is something I would love my daughter to read. Here's to all the amazing women being amazing!

Chapter 1: Take Off Your Cloak of Doubts

I use the phrase "cloak of doubts" because your self-doubt makes your potential and abilities invisible to yourself and the ones around you. We believe that we see an unsuccessful, loser, and ugly person in the mirror, but that is us (our own self) hiding under our cloak. The person inside waits to be found.

According to a widely known study from a Hewlett Packard internal report, men apply for employment even if they only meet 60% of the qualifications, but women only apply if they meet 100% of them. These occupations paid well and offered fantastic opportunities, but why did the women not apply? What was the loss at applying?

They were afraid of being "not qualified enough" and "being rejected" for the job. This was their self-doubt and lack of faith in themselves acting out. The effect of self-doubt is that we wait until we have checked all the boxes, maybe for too long, and then miss out on opportunities.

How many of you thought, "Should I speak up?" when you had an excellent idea in a meeting or a conversation you did not like in a family gathering and never actually said anything.

How often have you dressed up and felt beautiful, and someone pointed a degrading remark toward you, and your self-worth dropped to the floor?

It is time to believe in yourself and break free from self-doubts. Let's explore the roots of self-doubt.

1.1 What Hides Behind?

Self-doubters employ psychological strategies to maintain and sustain their negative attitude about themselves. They can be:

- **The Self-fulfilling Prophecy: "I can't."**

  "Our cerebral pathways eventually form patterns as a result of the way we speak to ourselves over time. If we tell ourselves things like "I'm a loser," "I'm not capable of doing this," or "I'm no good," these beliefs will gradually become engraved in our minds and become our reality. This type of thinking is based on two simple words: "I can't."

  When we believe we cannot, we put out less effort. After all, why to bother? We raise our expectancy of failure by putting in less effort, supporting our own negative ideas, and creating a vicious cycle.

- **The Impostor Syndrome: "I shouldn't."**

  Self-doubt is closely linked to the imposter syndrome. It shows the irrational sensation of being a sham, with luck-based accomplishments rather than genuine effort or skill. You believe that it will only be a matter of time before your actual self is revealed to others around you.

This imposter syndrome is frequently associated with despair and anxiety, and it can also be used to forecast these emotional difficulties. In other words, by putting your accomplishments in the hands of others, you are preventing yourself from understanding that you are just as deserving as everyone else.

- **Self-Sabotaging - "I didn't."**

It is tempting not to study at all if you are scared of failing a test. This way, if you fail, you will be able to blame it on not studying. It is clever to shift the blame from ourselves and place it on someone or something else. So, it was not you or your ability that let you down; it was the situation. You would have passed your test if you had studied. However, you failed because you did not study.

Fear of failure motivates self-sabotage. It is a procrastinator's dream. If you keep doing this for too long, you will end up with exactly what you were trying to prevent all along: When you attempt, you will start to feel you are incapable of success because you have forgotten how well you do.

- **A lack of self-compassion - "I'm a disaster."**

You are contributing to a broader problem with a lack of self-kindness by denying your own sense of accomplishment. While we are normally very helpful and loving to our friends in distress, we are considerably harsher on ourselves. According to research, Self-doubt has been linked to a lack of self-kindness. People who are friendly to themselves acknowledge their flaws rather than deny them and are better able to motivate themselves to improve. People who have a lot of self-doubts have a stronger need for approval from others. They are more concerned about negative feedback and failure, and they are tougher on themselves. All of this might lead to isolation.

Here is how you can tackle these psychological patterns.

1.2 Be Done with Doubts

Self-doubt is defined as a lack of belief in oneself and one's ability. It is an attitude that prevents you from achieving your goals and believing in yourself. Humility is a good character quality to have, but it is no longer useful if it is at your own expense. Let's look at strategies and habits to eliminate this destructive inner voice.

Identify and Replace Limiting Beliefs.

Your subconscious mind is responsible for 95% of your thoughts. That leaves only a small percentage of your choices to be deliberate.

Furthermore, in this part of your mind, your beliefs are created that you do not second-guess. Our values act as a road map for our lives. And your beliefs are mostly formed by the time you reach the age of seven. These beliefs that you learn as a youngster become so embedded in your brain that you do not question them, even if they differ from person to person.

We build the foundations of our views by assigning a feeling or emotion to individuals, circumstances, and prior events. As a result, your neurological system receives psychological cues from these beliefs, influencing your thoughts and interpreting your experiences. They connect your mind and body and your thoughts and habits. Follow these steps to avoid limiting your life:

- **Figure Out Your Limiting Beliefs.**

  What are some aspects of your life that you feel unsatisfactory with but are not actively attempting to improve? Do you feel secure when you think about your finances? Is your job secure, and does your pay support your living expenses? Are you in good health, and do you look for yourself and your body properly? How are your relationships? Are you enjoying your free time?

  I will give you an example from my own life. When I look through these aspects of my life, one that stands out as a challenge to me is how I spend my free time. To learn more about this, I would like to develop a list of my beliefs on leisure time. This is what it would look like:

  - I do not have time to enjoy myself.

  - Work should be prioritized over leisure.

  - People will think I am lazy if I enjoy time to myself.

> I should not be allowed to do the things I enjoy because I have a child.

- **Question Your Belief.**

What evidence do you have to back up your claim? Take, for example, the belief that no one likes you. Do you have people who are telling you this? Is it true that no one contacts you on your birthday or during the holidays? Do you have a difficult time getting along with your coworkers?

- **Consider Consequences of Your Belief.**

Consider the impact on your life if you hold this belief for the rest of your life. If you think that no one likes you, you are unlikely to make friends. This belief could become self-fulfilling, and you may find yourself spending most of your time alone. Feel the sadness at the thought of being cut off from others and the regret at having passed so many opportunities in life.

Consider yourself to be one of your friends. What would you say to yourself to persuade yourself that people like you? What concrete evidence would you offer? Try to see your belief through the eyes of an outsider, which means you should evaluate it objectively. What would you advise someone you love who was trying to set similar boundaries in their life?

Do not blindly follow your beliefs. Study them.

Say "No" to Being Powerless.

When being in victim mentality, we hold the belief that "nothing will make a difference." We get so stuck on our problems that we lose sight of the solutions. Even if someone offers us a solution, we may disregard it because we believe it will not work. That is why it is so hard for people who feel helpless to move out of their situation. They are unable to help themselves, and others are unable to help them as well. There are some strategies below to avoid being helpless and using your potential.

- **Accept the Problem**

  Do not waste time analyzing the situation, whining about it, or blaming someone for your misfortune when something negative or unexpected happens to you. This will not help to improve the problem. Accept the situation as it is instead. Surrendering entails accepting what is and trusting that things will improve. It is not the same as quitting, which many individuals do when they feel powerless.

- **Find What is Controllable**

  We always have some influence over most situations, even if we do not have complete control over everything. You have no power over the weather. It is impossible to stop the rain or the sun from shining. However, you can always get under a shade.

  The trick is to be aware of what you can and cannot control and to recognize the small window of control within the larger circle of uncontrollable factors. We stop feeling powerless when we focus on and take responsibility for the areas we have control over.

- **Take Whatever Small Step Possible**

Put your attention on what you do have control over and make tiny efforts toward your goals.

If you have lost your job, you would want to find another full-time career to replace your income. However, the hiring process can take a long time, and you have no say in whether or not a company hires you. You will eventually sink into insecurity and helplessness due to your decreasing savings if you simply remain at home all day waiting on the company to respond.

More opportunities may open up for you if you use your spare time to look for part-time or contract employment or even volunteer for a company.

It is depressing to focus on the perfect conclusion and then realize you do not have it right now. And the more you consider it, the worse it makes you feel. Rather than looking for a single answer to fix all of your problems at once, adopt small, consistent behaviors and let the solution reveal itself as you go.

For example, we may not be able to get out of the job we despise right now, but we may value the income we are receiving and set aside money each month to prepare for a career change. We may do our best every day to maintain a healthy relationship, even if we have no control over whether our spouse stays or goes. You do not always get what you want. However, you can always do something small right now to help yourself feel better about your situation.

Be open to suggestions. Instead of labeling and arguing why it might not work, find out if it does.

Cultivate Self-Compassion

Self-compassion is about realizing your needs and knowing and appreciating what you deserve. It is about making peace with who you are right now and being your most genuine self. It is about being easy on yourself and unconditionally loving yourself.

- **Give Yourself Grace**

  Does the butterfly look back at the caterpillar in shame?

  You need to be kind and extend grace to yourself. When you fall down, have grace. When you are ready to give up, when all you can see are your flaws and when you are at your lowest, be patient with yourself. Treat yourself with compassion. That is when you will really need it.

  You should accept where you are and who you are so you may make the most of it if you want to help yourself. It is fine to have a preference for what you want, but solely thinking of yourself worthy with only that goal achieved is not necessarily constructive.

- **Focus on Your Self Talk**

Positive self-talk is a type of self-care that you may practice just by choosing your thoughts. That means you can choose to think the opposite of your negative ideas when they arise. Instead of thinking, "I will never be able to do this," consider how you can adapt and improve by addressing problems. "I will do this one way or another, now or later."

Make a list of positive affirmations that are specific and purposeful. Make them powerful. Here's one to start with: if you are struggling with "enoughness" and do not feel like you are getting anywhere, simply say, "I am enough."

You will feel it, believe it, and live it, the more you say it or write it. This is true of all positive affirmations, and it affects how you treat yourself.

- **Do not Avoid Vulnerable Emotions**

Keep a journal of your feelings, rate your mood on a regular basis, and share it with someone you trust. Do not be frightened to seek support. You may have to confront your vulnerability as a result of this.

You are not weak if you are vulnerable. It enlightens you. In terms of how you relate to your emotions, you can use the RAIN technique or a mindfulness or meditation tool.

Here are the four steps in RAIN in a nutshell:

- ➢ R: Recognize what is happening

- ➢ A: Allow life to be just as it is

- ➢ I: Investigate inner experience

- ➢ N: Non-Identification

When you do not identify with a feeling but instead learn to think more rationally, you have accomplished non-identification. Emotional reasoning, a typical cognitive mistake in which you over-identify with emotions, is simple to fall into. It is possible that reality is not what you think it is.

Investing in self-care while cultivating self-compassion follows the three phases outlined above. You are treating yourself with compassion when you give yourself grace, anchor yourself with positive self-talk, and remain open to vulnerability.

Let Go of Perfectionism

Perfectionism is a self-destructive and compulsive belief system based on the thought that if I look flawless, live perfectly, and do everything precisely, I will be able to avoid or minimize the unpleasant feelings of humiliation, condemnation, and guilt.

Even though it is unattainable, you strive for it. It gives you the impression that you are in control. No, it is driving you.

- **Do Something Imperfectly on Purpose**

If you are a perfectionist or an overachiever, I am assuming just reading this step has made you feel uneasy! Why would you want to do things wrong on purpose?

It will help you get used to it. You cannot do everything flawlessly, and attempting to do so will drive you insane. You must develop the habit of performing at a below-average level.

I am not expecting you to go all out here. There is no reason to show up to a meeting with top management without having prepared or checking your PowerPoint for mistakes. Instead, choose a low-risk option. Consider taking a jewelry-making class. Arrive unprepared for a low-key encounter with a colleague. Play around with a new recipe. Work on a wacky Pinterest-inspired project. You will grow accustomed to being flawed - and you might even enjoy the process!

- **Perfection does not Define Your Self Worth**

While we think of ourselves in terms of perfection, we rarely think of the people we love in terms of perfection or imperfection. "I love you. You do not have to be perfect," we never say this to our children. We simply adore them, regardless of whether they are "perfect" or "imperfect."

It is not because we are blind to our loved ones' flaws; their value is not based on the concept of perfection.

Apply the same logic to yourself: your intrinsic worth is unrelated to your level of perfection.

- **Avoid Procrastinating**

Procrastination is an indication that you have a perfectionist mindset.

You are putting off your workout since you do not have an hour to spare. You do not have time to prepare a full week's worth of meals, so you skip meal prep. You do not meditate because it is difficult to sit for 20 minutes.

Ask yourself, "Am I avoiding this because I have an expectation of perfection?" the next time you find yourself postponing or putting something off that you know is vital for your health and self-care.

If you answer yes, there is a straightforward solution. Make a movc. Do anything. Just get started.

- **Consistency does not Require Perfection**

We all know that consistency is critical when it comes to long-term success. However, when we conflate consistency with perfection, we run into difficulty.

Consistency does not imply perfection or achievement on a daily basis. It entails showing up and performing the task most of the time. You should do it more often than you do not do it. That is all there is to it.

- **See Mistakes as Opportunities**

  Consider failure as a course correction when you fail—whether it is a modest failure at a new pastime you are trying out or a larger failure at work that others witness. When we start to turn off track, big or small, a failure becomes our teacher. The lessons we learn from our mistakes—whether in math class or in life—are usually the ones we remember the most because our mistakes stick with us.

  Furthermore, experiencing the disappointment of small to medium failures—and realizing that life goes on—will help us develop character and resilience for when we face larger-scale failure or actual difficulty later in life. Everyone faces hardships in life, from being laid off to losing a loved one prematurely, and having dealt with previous failures teaches us how to persevere in the face of adversity.

Not a single human on this planet is perfect. We are not made to be perfect. Strive for excellence, not perfection.

Work on Self-Awareness

One of the most effective personal growth resources you have is self-awareness. Make the most of it by figuring out what is causing your self-doubt. What circumstances set you off on a path of self-doubt? If there is a deficiency of competence in a particular area, resolve to address it. It could, for example, be a fear of giving presentations. It could also be a fear of failure. Whatever it is, work on it and prove to yourself that you can do it.

Beware of Your Close Circle

According to popular belief, we are the average of the five individuals with whom we spend the most time. We do not have any scientific study to back up this claim, but it does include a seed of truth. The people we spend most of our life with can have a huge impact on us. Experiences change neuronal networks in the brain, according to brain plasticity research. According to Dr. John Kounios, professor of brain science and psychology, our neural connections change even after a 20-minute talk! Who are the people you are around most of your time? What impact do you think they have on you? Do you leave feeling better or worse about yourself after spending time with them?

Here are six symptoms that your friendship is causing you to lose your confidence.

- You do not feel you can express yourself when you are together. If your friend responds to what you are saying with an insensitive tone that makes you want to restrain yourself, consider it a red flag. Your self-confidence will gradually decline if you are unable to speak about the things in which you believe.

- No two friends are at the exact same point in their lives, whether professionally or personally. However, that should never come between you and your friendship. Is your friend bragging about their accomplishments to the point where it sounds like they are taunting you?

- You are worried that you are putting them in a bad light in front of their friends and relatives.

Friends who are judgmental and condemning are the ones who will make you feel inferior. The lower your self-esteem becomes around this friend, the more likely you will feel that you do not belong to their friends, as if you cannot keep up with their exciting lives.

- You ignore their SMS and calls when you do not have anything exciting to say. The best friendships are ones in which you do not feel obligated to put on a show. You can just be yourself and believe that they will accept you for who you are.

- You feel hesitant shopping for clothes with them or mentioning your weight or size. It could be an indication that they make you feel bad about yourself just because of the way you look. Believe me, this is a projection of their own security and has nothing to do with you. Your appearance does not define your self-worth. Give nobody the power to define your self-worth.

Respect yourself enough to realize when it is time to leave a room.

Find Validation from Within

Your employer compliments you on your most recent project. Your term paper receives an A. Your significant other compliments you on your appearance. These are examples of external validation or affirmation from a source other than yourself. However, the issue occurs when we begin to rely on others to make life decisions and determine our self-worth.

If your personality development continues in this direction, you will never feel secure in your decisions or in yourself. You will be on the lookout for someone to give you permission to do things that affect your life.

- **Become Aware**

  Recognize your need for external validation and think about where it might come from. Where has this need not been met in your life? When have you not felt good enough in your life, or what has happened in your past that has made you feel insufficient?

  Consider your early life experiences and connections with family members, as these are the foundations of self-esteem.' Simply put, if you are aware that you are looking for validation from others, you will be more likely to notice when you are doing it and subsequently cut it down.

- **Focus on Your Behavior**

  The rest of the intervention you want to undertake is all behavioral. You should look at what behaviors you do to get validation - whether it is posting photographs on social media or making statements to draw compliments from other people. Find ways to cut down on this behavior.

  You may feel happy in the short term by receiving validation from others, or, in other situations, you may be extremely disappointed because you do not receive the validation you desire.

- **Work on Self Esteem**

  It is a sure sign you have weak self-esteem if you are looking for other people's acceptance. That is why this is one of the most critical issues to address. The only way to boost your self-esteem, in the long run, is to live a life that makes you proud of your actions. You may achieve this by standing up for yourself and putting yourself in positive situations. It is also about taking pride in how you live your life. Self-esteem is about how you treat yourself and the decisions you make in your life, like how you let others treat you, what you avoid, and what you attract into your life.

- **Look at Your Strengths**

  Examining your recent accomplishments and recognizing your abilities is one technique to help you boost your self-esteem.

  You would not be brilliant at everything; no one is, but there will be things you enjoy doing and feel confident in your ability to do. The road to confidence and self-belief begins when you can pinpoint these and do them successfully without the assistance or validation of others.

You need to hold on to and love the little part of yourself that whispers, "You are capable" when times are hard.

Be Skeptical of your Thoughts

Self-doubt is not a character flaw. It is nothing more than a mental habit.

All-day long, our brains bombard us with thoughts. For example, "Remember to pick up milk on the way home." Some are unhelpful, such as "Why do I have to be so stupid all the time!"

You should not allow your self-doubt to get the best of you. It is just an unintentionally reinforced cognitive pattern that has become a habit. So, it is just a habit. And habits are always reversible.

Try to develop a healthy skepticism of your own ideas. It is not true that it is true just because you have an idea.

If you make it a habit to question your own thoughts—especially the ones that are not very useful, like chronic self-doubt—you will be able to take away their power over you.

Avoid Self-Criticism

Your private inner dialogue can be a great stepping stone or a big roadblock to achieving your personal and professional objectives. Your self-talk will drain your mental power if you regularly make negative predictions like "I'm going to mess up" or call yourself names. So here's how to avoid it:

- **Write it Down**

   The majority of our self-criticism occurs in our head. It takes the shape of negative self-talk, and it repeats itself in our heads.

   The issue is that thoughts move very fast. Because we are all capable of thinking so quickly, we can have a ton of self-critical thoughts in just a few moments. Sadly, all these thoughts trigger a painful emotion, such as anxiety or despair, so being self-critical in your thinking can quickly provoke to a lot of negative emotions.

Pull out a notebook and write your critical thoughts down whenever you find yourself getting mean to yourself and self-criticizing. This has two major advantages:

1. It will cause you to slow down. You would not be able to write as quickly as you can think. You will feel a lot better if you only have 6 negative thoughts rather than 60.

2. It offers you a sense of perspective. In our heads, even the most nonsensical beliefs can appear incredibly persuasive and real. However, when those thoughts are written down, their illogical or extreme character becomes more obvious.

- **Find Logic**

The content of self-criticism is often inaccurate or unrealistic for persons who battle with chronic self-criticism. You punish yourself irrationally. This manifests as cognitive distortions, as defined by psychologists. Distorted self-criticism, like funhouse mirrors that distort your image to appear as abnormally tiny or overweight, can make you appear (and feel) very worthless or incompetent.

- **Learn to Get Rejected**

  When we are surprised or ambushed by a circumstance, we often become highly critical of ourselves.

  For example, before going into a meeting with your boss to discuss a new idea, you can think to yourself, "My boss frequently changes her mind about projects. I am guessing she will come up with some reason not to go ahead with this new concept. It doesn't mean it is a bad idea or that she would not eventually accept it. That is just how she thinks about things."

  When your boss inevitably criticizes your concept, you will be prepared because you have expected it and are prepared. It will make it less likely that you will be caught off guard and that your habit of self-criticism will kick in.

  In other words, removing the element of surprise from triggers of self-criticism reduces the likelihood of extensive self-criticism.

- **Criticism is not a Motivator**

  We use self-criticism as motivation, which is one of the main reasons behind chronic self-criticism. Those who are extremely hard on themselves frequently perform even worse because their attention and energy are spent on self-criticism. You are more likely to succeed in the future if you learn to be more kind to yourself and self-compassionate, particularly after mistakes.

Cherish your strengths and accomplishments and work towards improvement with kindness.

These are some strategies that will help you put your self-doubt behind you.

Chapter 2: Adorn Yourself with Confidence

Amelia Earhart was the first woman ever to fly alone across the Atlantic Ocean. During that period in history, Amelia Earhart was one of the many extremely skilled female pilots at that time. Although she was talented, I do not believe it was the reason for her success. Rather, it was her self-confidence, desire to do the impossible, and belief in her ability to succeed. Confidence is just as important as competence since it leads to attention, action, and resilience, which Amelia demonstrated on her transatlantic trip.

According to Pauline Claunce and Suzanne Imes' female confidence challenge, women regularly remark that they do not believe they deserve their jobs and that they are "imposters" who could be discovered at any time. According to the study, women are more concerned about being hated, outshining others, appearing unattractive, or attracting too much attention.

According to a Cornell University study, men overestimate their abilities and performance, whereas women underestimate both. There is no difference in quantity or quality in their actual performance.

So if women have the same abilities as men, what do they lack? Confidence in their abilities. Let's study a bit more about what self-confidence can add to your life.

2.1 Does it Matter?

Confidence is the belief that our actions will result in a positive outcome. In other words, when we are confident, we believe, we are good enough and have something valuable to contribute. Those beliefs motivate us to take action, such as applying for a job, maintaining our relationship standards, trying something new on our own, asking for a promotion, or moving to a new place.

- **Self-Esteem Boost**

  When you have self-confidence, you start to value yourself and everything you can do and place yourself in a positive light.

  You form a protective shield around yourself with your self-confidence. People will respect you just because of how you have presented yourself when speaking with them.

  You learn that you do not take anything less than you deserve because you already know that you are worth it. It will also help you find the right person for you and establish a healthy and long-term relationship with the one you deserve.

- **Advocating for Yourself**

  You can defend yourself in any scenario if you have self-confidence. You will be able to talk for yourself as well. People may treat you the way they want if you lack confidence, which can be upsetting. All that matters when you have strong self-esteem is how you see yourself. How others perceive you does not matter. You free yourself from fear of judgement.

You have the ability to rise above fear, whether it is fear of the unknown or you are scared of what other people might think of you. You can also deal with any circumstance that most people avoid.

It also enables you to manage your emotions and understand how to act ethically. You can also impact what people think and how they act.

- **Keeping the Spark Alive with Your Partner**

One of the keys to keeping your spouse interested in you is maintaining your self-confidence. You will become highly attractive if you have a high level of self-confidence. You understand what you want from life and in your relationship, and you will work hard to achieve it. This makes you self-sufficient and appealing, qualities that men admire in women.

- **People Looking Up to You**

You can become a role model for others if you have self-confidence. People will want to associate with you.

You start to see the bright side of everything and believe that nothing is truly impossible.

When you have high self-confidence, you will place a greater emphasis on self-love and self-esteem. You will also have a better awareness of yourself and be able to properly identify your flaws.

You are more likely to be successful in your work, relationship, and life with high self-confidence.

2.2 Glow with Confidence

Self-assurance is linked to nearly every aspect of a happy and fulfilling existence. When you claim that you have complete confidence in someone, you imply that you have complete faith in them. Similarly, self-confidence entails believing in oneself and one's skills. It is the ability to feel at ease in a variety of situations while keeping loyal to yourself. It is believing in oneself while accepting and improving one's weaknesses. The definition of self-confidence is made up of all of these descriptions taken together. Here's how you can build your self-confidence:

Find the Root Cause

Finding the source of low self-confidence can lead to a road map for increasing positive self-confidence. Self-reflection and journaling are important steps to start. Try this exercise to figure out what is causing your low self-confidence:

- Make a list of any low self-confidence phrases or thoughts that come up for you over a week.

- "Who or what told you that?" question yourself for each negative thought.

- Decide if you want to give that voice authority over you.

- Create a plan of action to go forward by writing down how you can solve the situation.

Figure out the reason behind your low confidence and address it.

Find out What Confidence Feels Like

Take some time to notice how you feel in your body when you are confident. "How will you know when you have reached a satisfactory level of self-confidence?" is a great question to consider. At work, you might need to be more assertive. Maybe you need to wear the clothes you have desired to wear for a long time. You might even approach your crush and introduce yourself. This will differ from one person to the next. As a result, no one else needs to understand it.

Design Your Ideal Life

Do you know accomplishing your goals boosts your confidence? So why not work towards a life you want and are proud of?

Make a list of everything you want to do in as many different aspects of your life as possible. Consider the following:

> **Your Personal Life:** Would you prefer to relocate, improve, or expand your current residence? Where in the world would you love to live if you could live anywhere?

Have you always desired to travel to a specific country or region? Would you like to take a vacation across the world? Would you like to travel across the world while working?

> **Your work:** Consider whether you are content in your current job or whether you have always wanted to do something else, such as establish your own business or make a living by painting, writing, or practicing another creative skill.

> **Your Family:** Are there any connections in your immediate or extended family that you would like to improve? Would you like to remain single if you are single, or do you have a long-term goal to marry and have children?

Write down everything that comes to mind. Concentrate on your deepest wishes, dreams, and objectives, no matter how irrational or unattainable they may appear. Admit that these are the things you truly desire in life.

Next, imagine how your life will be once you have accomplished your long-term objectives.

- **Visualize Your Goals**

    It is equally crucial to picture your fulfilled dreams on paper and visualize them in your thoughts.

    Find images that represent your aspirations, cut them out, and put them together in a collage. You might also construct a digital scrapbook or paste photographs into a scrapbook. Along with the photographs, write about your goals. Include motivational phrases and anything else that will motivate you to keep going.

- **Break Down Goals**

Picking a tiny, measurable milestone is one of the most effective setting methods. Break down everything you wish to alter about your job, personal, or family life into smaller goals and be specific.

If your long-term aim is to save money for a house, your first goal might be to save $1,000 in the coming three months. Decide what it means to be healthier if that is your goal. It could entail eating two servings of veggies every day for the next month or going for a five-times-per-week stroll.

Let's go above the $1,000 objective again in the next three months. What method will you use to do this?

> Over the course of a month, write down/figure out all of the areas where you spend money (or several months).

> After taxes, write down how much money you make each month.

> You will need to save $333 per month to save $1,000 in three months.

> Examine all of your spending habits and identify areas where you may save money.

> Determine whether there are any possibilities for you to generate extra money in the coming months if that is possible.

Although the list may appear daunting, keep in mind that you do not have to complete all of the tasks at once. It is critical to master the art of concentration if you want to achieve your goal.

- **Schedule Your Tasks**

Consult your calendar once you have completed your entire list. Schedule each task. You will review your expenditures on Tuesday at 2 p.m. You will examine your sources of income on Thursday at 7 p.m. Take it one step at a time as you work through the list.

Scheduling each job is an excellent approach to keeping track of your big to-do list. What you have to do when the clock ticks 2 p.m. on a Tuesday is one thing. You should not worry about the remaining steps. You have already determined when you will complete each one.

- **Celebrate Your Wins**

Treat yourself to a small reward whenever you complete a big milestone on your path to reaching your long-term goals. It may be a day trip, a book you have been meaning to read, or anything else that makes you happy.

It is absolutely essential to be kind to yourself and appreciate the journey as much as you enjoy your life once you arrive.

Even if you do not achieve your ideal life for some time, the steps that bring you closer to it will make you confident and happy. Small wins go a long way. Enjoy the process.

Learn to Love Your Body

Negative body image should not be overlooked. Its effects can have a profound physical and mental impact on the body. People suffering are frequently preoccupied with the image of the "ideal body," to the point where they forget what is healthy and establish unreasonable objectives for themselves, leading to additional mental discomfort and disappointment. Women are the worst offenders for not accepting and loving their bodies. Approximately 91 percent of women are unhappy with their bodies, according to the charity DoSomething.org, and more than 40 percent of women and around 20 percent of men said they would consider cosmetic surgery in the future.

Trade negative for positive; everything, not just your thoughts. Avoid certain friends or family members who only have bad things to say or make hurtful statements to you. Surround yourself with individuals that are rooting for you and just want what is best for you. People that radiate negativity and nastiness are insecure people who say hurtful things to make themselves feel better.

Make new friends who are enjoyable to be around and who will not judge you. Getting out and socializing can give you a significant boost in confidence. I will discuss body positivity in detail in the next chapter.

Adopt a Growth Mindset

A growth mindset motivates you to look beyond your current abilities and knowledge, constantly seeking methods to improve. Simply substituting the word "yet" for "I'm not confident," the old belief becomes "I'm not confident yet." This includes the condition of learning new skills in order to gain confidence.

Here are some helpful hints:

- You must first believe in yourself. Use a mantra daily. Tell yourself that you are capable of any change you wish. It may take some effort to help you believe it, but you can do it by reminding yourself of the benefits - accomplishment, and growth.

- Avoid blaming other People or your shortcomings on how the situation was. You should accept responsibility for who you are and for maximizing your natural talents and abilities. Take a moment the next time you find yourself blaming something or someone, accept responsibility, discover the lesson, and move on.

- Those looking for change must be curious as well. Not knowing is a source of pleasure rather than dread or humiliation. Ask inquiries and look for further information to follow up on it.

- Give yourself permission to fail. It is critical that you attempt and fail and then try and fail again, as hard as it may be. Every failure is a stepping stone toward achievement. I am sure I do not need to remind you of the numerous notable people who failed badly before becoming leaders, influencers, and role models.

People generally talk about their accomplishments because we live in a failure-averse culture. Don't you occasionally get to hear about people's failure stories? Understanding that failure is inevitable, and part of the life experience will enable you to live more freely.

- Get comfortable functioning out of your comfort zone. For a lot of us, the comfort zone is a haven. It is a place where we may be free of stress. "Free from problems" does not imply "free from growth." Push yourself to new heights.

- Do not put too much focus on outcomes. Sure, outcomes are important but do not forget to congratulate yourself on your efforts. Self-praise for a valiant effort might keep you going for a long time. When things get rough, it is all about the process.

- Be wary of jealousy. When confronted with someone else's success, think to yourself, "I will use their success as a model for what I want to achieve," rather than " I wish I had achieved what they have." The former motivates you to succeed, while the latter restricts you. Praise yourself for helping you on your way to achievement.

- Finally, do not let your ego's defense stand in the way of making adjustments that will make you happier and more successful. A growth attitude will force you to explore areas where you are less at ease, more afraid, and less accomplished. The ego does not like this, yet giving in to it leads to mediocrity. If you want to succeed, you must be willing to confront your ego, limiting beliefs, and perceived limits.

Do not let your fixed mindset fix your life as it is.

Treat Emotions as Temporary

Emotions are similar to tunnels. To see the light at the end, you must first travel through the darkness.

There is a beginning, a middle, and an end to emotions. Emotions can be overwhelming at times, but they are only temporary. At their most basic level, emotions are biological reactions to stimuli in your environment. If your internet goes out right before your presentation, you can have a panic attack. You can be filled with delight if you receive a surprise delivery from your sister. If you receive a text from your ex, you may experience a wave of grief. Whatever the stimulus and corresponding emotion, they are all data points that will help you decide what to do next.

In terms of confidence, any feeling that is preventing you from taking action, such as stress, anxiety, or fear, is just transitory. Once the storm has passed, you can plan your next move. As the cliché says, "Feel the fear and do it regardless."

Photoshop Your Self Image

Our self-image is extremely important to us, far more than we know. We have a mental image of ourselves that determines our level of self-assurance. It is about how you feel about yourself, your personality, and your abilities. However, this picture is not set in stone. You have the ability to alter it.

So, if your hopes and goals include obtaining the perfect job, being promoted, or becoming a successful entrepreneur, you must ensure that your self-image matches your thoughts.

Your self-image is built on your self-beliefs, and if what you want does not align with those beliefs, getting the result you want will be much more difficult.

If you believe you are not good enough, do not have what it takes to be successful, or do not deserve to earn a lot of money, thinking and desiring it would not make it happen because your self-perception is far more powerful and deeply ingrained in your subconscious than any passing notion.

Focus and determination are admirable qualities, but are they enough to overcome your beliefs? Because if your beliefs are how you identify yourself, they are a part of your identity. Changing how you think of yourself would mean changing how you define yourself. It will trip you up time and time again if what you desire is not in accordance with who you are.

So, if you are trying to make changes in your life, in any area, and you are having trouble doing so, consider your self-image. Is your self-perception "in line" with your desired outcomes and level of success?

Work on your self-image and use your mental photo-shopping skills. If it is not very good, replace it. Figure out why you perceive yourself in that light and how to change it.

Boost Competency

Our self-esteem improves as we improve ourselves. In some ways, when we stop learning, we begin to die. We must find ways to increase our competency on a daily basis, regardless of what degree we have obtained or what initials follow our name. Let's get started.

- **Learn Something New**

  Let's start with some self-development activities that can assist you in developing new skills:

  - Taking an online course is a fantastic opportunity to pick up new skills, broaden your horizons, and grow. There are so many excellent free online courses available in any skill you want to learn.

  - Learning an instrument can be a wonderful opportunity to connect with like-minded people, find a healthy outlet for emotional expression, and cultivate a lifelong interest.

  - Learning a new language is an excellent way to improve your skills, learn about a different culture, and expand your horizons. Learning a new language can also provide you with new travel chances and connect you to a large number of new potential friends.

  - Start a business. Freelancing, consulting, and online teaching are just a few examples of the types of businesses you can start.

- **Improve Your Habits**

Motivation is a fuel propelling you forward. It is your habits that keep you going. So, let's look at some ways to improve yourself by changing your habits.

> - Successful people exercise on a regular basis for a reason. It helps us stay focused and motivated by boosting our immune systems, giving us greater energy, and regulating our hormones and emotions. Consider working out with a friend, downloading an exercise app, or making a daily goal, no matter how little, if you want to start exercising frequently.
>
> - Many of the world's most successful people regard reading as a daily means of self-improvement. Bill Gates, for example, reads 50 books every year, or nearly one every week.
>
> - With so many harmful choices available, it can be difficult to eat healthily in today's world. On the other hand, our diets have a significant impact on our happiness, well-being, and success. Start small and focus on consistency while trying to break a negative habit. Start by eating at least three different types of fresh fruits and vegetables every day.

> ➢ "You are what you eat," as the cliché goes, applies to everything we consume, including what we listen to and see. Every movie and podcast influences our mental and emotional states, and we listen to social media posts. Indeed, according to a new study, social media has a negative impact on one's well-being and increases feelings of loneliness and depression. So, listen to some encouraging podcasts or watch some motivational and educational television.

> ➢ Spend some time in nature with yourself, sitting quietly and watching the sunset. Just be. This can be really unsettling at first. However, learning to be alone with yourself without distractions is an important aspect of significant self-development.

- **Improve Your Focus**

The ability to direct your attention to where you want it to go without being distracted by external stimuli, unpleasant emotions or bad habits is known as focus. So, here are some self-improvement techniques to help you focus better.

> ➢ Create a strategy and schedule time to work on your wishes so you can turn them into goals. To-do list apps can come in handy.

> ➢ Meditate. It can help you:

>> o Encourage emotional well-being.

- o Increase your attention span.

        - o Improve your self-awareness.

        - o Boost your sleep quality.

        - o Reduce the effects of aging on memory.

        - o Control pain.

    - ➢ Keep a journal. According to research, expressing your thoughts and feelings in this way can help to:

        - o Reduce the symptoms of arthritis, asthma, and other health problems.

        - o Boost your immune system.

        - o Enhance your cognitive abilities.

        - o Minimize detrimental consequences of stress.

It is also a fantastic strategy to keep on track with your objectives while simultaneously increasing your feelings of gratitude and happiness.

- **Manage Your Emotions**

You will not get too far if you are unable to handle your distressing emotions, no matter how smart you are. Below are some strategies for dealing with your emotions.

> Keep an eye on your emotional reactions because they can quickly overwhelm us and compel us to act in ways we would not otherwise. As a result, self-improvement requires learning to recognize your emotions and regulate your behaviors.

> Work on your fear of failure. On the opposite side, fear and your comfort zone are everything you have ever desired. Consider working on conquering your fear of failure if you want to develop yourself. Try Noah Kagan's coffee challenge to get started. This accomplished entrepreneur recommends going into a coffee shop and asking for a 10% discount for no reason, then waiting for a response. He guarantees you will learn something about yourself that will surprise you.

> Think of healthy ways to express yourself. Music, art, athletics and literature, are just a few of the various ways to express your feelings.

- **Improve Your Relationships**

The status of our relationships has a significant impact on our overall well-being. So, here are some self-improvement strategies to help you enjoy your relationships while making yourself better.

> Find ways to meet new people. This will not only allow you to improve your social skills, but it will also expose you to new perspectives on the world. Find fresh ways to meet new individuals who will encourage and motivate you. Consider joining a yoga studio- a local gym class, if you wish to enhance your fitness.

> What behaviors in your relationship should you improve? Perhaps you can spend more time with people you care about and listen to them rather than speaking to them?

> Maintain Boundaries. Our relationships, eventually our lives, are shaped by our boundaries (or lack thereof). Is there something you wish someone had not done? How would you approach this situation with compassion?

We feel abused and mistreated when we fail to set limits and hold individuals accountable. This is why sometimes we attack who they are when we should address a choice or behavior. Realize that it is much more hurtful.

The more competent you are, the more self-assured you will be.

Face Your Fears

Stop putting off things like asking someone out on a date or applying for a promotion until you are more confident. Facing your fears head-on is one of the most effective strategies to boost your confidence in these situations.

Even if you are scared that you will embarrass yourself or make a mistake, give it a shot. Furthermore, a little self-doubt can improve performance. Think of it as just a test and see what happens.

You could discover that making a few errors or being nervous is not as bad as you thought. And with each step forward, you gain more faith in yourself. Finally, this can help you avoid taking risks that will have serious negative consequences.

Find Solutions

When you find solutions for your problems instead of dwelling on them, you will learn to have faith in yourself. No matter how complex the problem is, you will trust yourself to deal with it. Solving your problems on your own will give you a confidence boost. It will, in turn, help you solve more problems making it a positive cycle.

Here are five pointers to help you improve your problem-solving skills and become more efficient.

- **Define the Problem**

  If you had an hour to address a problem, you would spend 55 minutes thinking about the issue and 5 minutes thinking about solutions.

It may appear straightforward, but many problems stay unsolvable because a deliberate effort to truly grasp and define the problem has not been made. Consider how you used to feel when you were in school. Have you ever approached a teacher for help with a question you were having trouble answering, and they immediately gave you a solution? Most likely not. Instead, they likely went over the question with you and discussed what it really was that you were asking to make sure you were working on the right problem.

- **Address the Problem Behind a Problem**

Before you start implementing solutions, you need to look at the situation from every angle. Consider if there are any other issues that are causing this problem. If this is the case, you must address it first. You might get tunnel vision when you are tackling a problem, yet there are usually several factors at play. Zoom out from the current situation and see all of the contributing reasons to the problem.

- **Brainstorm Solutions**

The initial idea that comes to mind might not be the finest, but the more you concentrate, the more options you will find. So, brainstorming all possible ideas is an important part of problem-solving.

It is good to think about the "perfect solution" as you brainstorm. Defining your final goal will help you come up with new ideas for how to get there.

- **Pick a Solution**

  You should be able to choose which solution is the most beneficial for your problem. Compare the outcome of the solutions you consider to be the most desirable. Which is the best option for you in the current situation?

- **Prepare If It Fails**

  Consider the consequences of the solution before solving your problem with the best-fit solution. Now is the moment to start thinking about the worst-case scenarios– What happens if the solution does not work? If you know what you will do, you will be able to plan effectively for it. Even if you lose at first, you will learn something. Do not think of it as a failure.

- **Set Deadline**

  Create a timeline for your solution. Determine when you will put the solution in place, how long it will take to complete, and when you will see results.

  What steps do you need to reach this deadline?

  It is critical to set a deadline and establish criteria for measuring achievement. How will you know if you are making progress or not? How will you compare this solution's outcome to the outcome of another?

  Set a series of short-term reporting deadlines. Consider which key performance indicators will allow you to monitor the achievement of your outcomes.

A big part of taking charge of your life is to solve your problems on your own.

Look for a Role Model

Ideally, it should be someone you regularly encounter, such as a coworker, a family member, or a friend - someone who has a lot of confidence and whom you want to follow. Observe them and pay attention to how they act. What do they say and when, how do they move, how do they speak? When faced with a difficulty or a mistake, how do they react? What are their social interactions like, and how do others react to them?

If you get the opportunity, speak with them to understand more about how they think and what motivates them.

Speaking with self-assured people and being around with them will usually make you feel more self-assured. Learn from people who have accomplished the tasks and goals you want to do, and allow their confidence to reflect on you.

These strategies will help you hold your head high and feel confident.

Chapter 3: Embrace Yourself with Love

In our society, women feel constantly pressured to look a specific way, feel a specific way, and act a specific way. Our life choices are constantly criticized and questioned. We are made to feel like we are not enough no matter what we do. I ask you to think about one thing. When everybody around you is unfair to you, the last thing you need is you attacking yourself too. The meaner everybody else is to you, the fiercer you need to love yourself. It is extremely hard to do when you feel the pressure defining you. But know that you owe it to yourself to consider yourself worthy of all good things. Your body and mind are unique, making their beauty unmatchable.

Perfection is the lowest standard. Being true to yourself is what matters.

Let's discuss the idea of "perfect" a bit more and why it is absurd.

3.1 Am I Normal?

Perfect is the new normal. We do everything in our life, striving for this "normal."

We all have our "perfect" scripted responses—I am doing fantastic! Work is fantastic! Yes, I have got it all figured out!

We might pass them out when we catch up with a buddy or welcome a coworker in the morning. Alternatively, thanks to social media, we may communicate the same message without saying anything. We share our ideal breakfast, a snug night in straight from a William Sonoma catalog, or a Bachelor-level romantic night.

It was something I used to do all the time. I would post three times a day on Instagram to show off my perfect existence. The job! What a lovely city! The total bliss that lasts 24 hours a day, seven days a week! Look at that: avocado toast! Is not it fantastic? And how did I respond when friends inquired about my well-being? I always reacted with a resounding Great!

However, a few months after graduating from college, I began to notice a significant disparity between the life I projected to people and my actual existence. I felt as if I were balancing myself on the edge of a cliff. On the one hand, I had a perfect existence that I had documented and shared with the rest of the world. On the other hand, my reality was studded with happy moments but also dense with obstacles and personal difficulties.

I felt like I was living a false life and contributing to the pressure we all feel to be "perfect." We need to stop giving in the pressure to be perfect and put this pressure on others too.

When I started to drop my guard around other people, I discovered a whole new universe of wonderful conversations. Friends on Instagram whom I followed, began to disclose that they did not have it all together, either-even if their accounts suggested otherwise. Knowing I was not alone, I began to let go of the "perfect" pressure I had acquired from so many people.

But what was the best part of talking about my problems with others? It allowed me to build an army of people who could assist me. For example, when I shared my struggles at work, it instantly opened the door for someone else to share theirs. Then it was only natural to inquire about how that individual handled it all, to get their advice on pushing through or dealing with problems head-on. I realized I had a lot of people in my corner who could help me with suggestions and advice. All I had to do was break free from my "It's going fantastic!" attitude and admit that I needed help.

I want to help you be "you." So let's begin.

3.2 Give Yourself a Warm Hug

We often set unrealistically high standards for ourselves because society expects us to be perfect. We have a tendency to forget that everyone, including those we consider to be flawless, have imperfections.

Self-acceptance and self-love are essential components of happiness and good health. We cut ourselves off from the energy that keeps us alive when we refuse to accept ourselves.

When we do not accept ourselves as we are, we are, in essence, exhausting ourselves on the inside. And guess who loses when we fight against ourselves? It is critical to acknowledge that we all have weaknesses. Everyone makes mistakes from time to time. Making mistakes is not something you should avoid at all costs. It is one of the most effective ways to learn and develop.

Accepting our talents and shortcomings and reconciling the opposing aspects of our inner world is essential for our health and happiness. Plus, you would not be able to accomplish anything in the outside world unless you first address your inner world. Below are some strategies for you to work towards self-acceptance and self-love.

Practice True Self-Love

There is no finish point to when you officially love yourself. Self-love is neither permanent nor consistent. We frequently define love in a fairytale way, in which everything must be flawless, and then apply the same pressure to self-love, which is unrealistic. Commitment, endurance, acceptance, or general neutrality are sometimes all it takes to love ourselves, just as it is with other long-term partnerships. Continue reading for these helpful hints on how to truly love oneself.

- **Accept Yourself**

  We must first acknowledge our realities before we can embrace our flawed selves. What we resist, continues to exist. In other words, denying what's going on increases your chances of engaging in negative self-talk ("It should not be this way" or "I should not have done that"). You will be better able to accept and move past the things you cannot control if you practice acknowledging your reality in nonjudgmental words ("This is my situation" or "This is what happened"). Acceptance is crucial here; you do not have to enjoy what is going on. It is natural to be disappointed if you were not called back for a second interview, but recognizing the facts of the situation ("They didn't call me back, and I'm disappointed") might help you avoid feeling disappointment. Instead of repeatedly beating yourself for what you should have done differently, the goal is to validate your ideas and feelings first, then practice self-acceptance to avoid being lost in a self-blame cycle.

- **Stick to the Facts**

Suffering is represented by Buddhists as two arrows. The first arrow represents an unfortunate event that occurred to us — an arrow that was hurtful and beyond our control. The second arrow represents the story we tell ourselves about what happened — this is self-inflicted misery. Self-love is not shooting ourselves with the second arrow.

For example, the first arrow may be the death of a loved one due to COVID-19. The second arrow may be that you convince yourself that they would not have died if you could just get them to the doctor sooner.

- **Recognize that Healing Takes Time**

If you are from a minority or historically oppressed group, you might internalize messages that suggest you are unimportant. Even if you do not feel the statements about your particular group are true about you, there may be pressure to perform above expectations in order to disprove them. In the effort to prove their worth and deserving of respect on an exterior level, some people begin to neglect their emotional, physical, and mental requirements.

It can also be difficult for trauma survivors to believe they are deserving of love because they are typically plagued by feelings of shame and self-blame. We must recognize that overcoming oppression and trauma can be quite difficult.

What does it mean to you to honor your body? Self-care staples include having a warm bath with scented candles or essential oils, cueing up some of your favorite tunes, and dancing it out in your living room. On the other hand, your body-centered kindness does not have to look like that. For example, going for a walk, eating a good meal, or wearing comfy pants can be more tempting to you.

- **Practice Boundaries**

In order to cultivate self-love, it is crucial to set healthy limits in partnerships. Avoid spending time and energy with those that make you feel unworthy, such as parents, friends, or partners. If you cannot stop all communication right away or at all (say, with a demanding boss or a strict parent), try practicing radical acceptance and setting even small boundaries, such as not checking your emails in the evening or ending a phone conversation with a loved one who is bringing you down.

You show others how it is okay to love you by the kind of love you extend towards yourself.

Redefine Happiness

According to research in the field of positive psychology, a happy person is someone who feels regular good feelings like joy, pride, and interest, as well as infrequent (but not nonexistent) negative emotions like sadness, worry, and rage. Positive emotions do not imply the absence of unpleasant emotions, which is the key to these definitions. A "happy person" goes through the same range of emotions as everyone else, but the frequency with which they go through the bad ones may be different.

Happiness can also be defined as a certain joyful feeling you experience while you are young. You may feel the happiness at that moment and whenever you think back on it.

That time was a summer day, and I was running barefoot on the scorching cement two doors down from my best friend Ethan's house. I would run as quickly as I could, hopping from grass to cement, pretending the pavement was lava — which one could argue it was, given the scorching temperatures — in an attempt to cool my tingling feet. I could feel my heart beating. The wind was blowing my curls away from my face. The buildup was the beginning of my euphoria, but it was not until I sneaked into his house, put a finger to my lips, told his mother not to give me away, and ran into his room and jumped on him that I became truly happy. I always succeeded in terrifying him, and then we would both laugh and eat hot fudge sundae downstairs while planning what mischief we would get up to that day.

I was not concerned with the number of calories in the hot fudge sundae or whether Ethan was busy and would be offended by my actions. Instead, I was letting go of everything, which allowed me to find true happiness. Even remembering the memory brings me back to a good place.

As we get older, everyone around us, including our parents, teachers, and the media, advise us to live a happy life and we must accomplish the following: We have to go to school and possibly learn stuff we do not care about because they earn money, and we need money to support our families. We must also perform generous deeds, not because of the goodness of our hearts, but because it will make us appear to be a better person, which will lead to greater opportunities and happiness! Are you starting to notice a pattern?

Finally, we put our passions, dreams, and desires in a box deep inside the crevices of our minds and pursue the path that is taught to us every day to achieve the final goal: this supposed "happiness." How can anybody be happy if he is a slave, slave to happiness' pursuit?

We should let go, just as we did as children, rather than focusing on the illusion of "the route to happiness." Our goal should be to pursue our passions and enjoy life, and happiness will arrive at some point along the way. If happiness is your primary goal, you will not be able to accomplish it.

Stop with the Comparison

It is hard not to compare yourself to others on social media. Your body is not fit enough, your clothes are not fashionable enough, and your home is not big enough. It may even make you feel as though you are not good enough. Comparisons rob us of our happiness, our earnings, and our sanity. We will end up draining all of our energy trying to keep up if we do not quit comparing ourselves to others! We must interrupt the cycle of comparison because it is a game we will never win.

- **Find Confidence in Your Strengths**

    Though it is tough to ignore when someone else is better than you at something, there are always things you excel in. To prevent comparison, you should start focusing on your strengths.

    Start jotting down things you enjoy about yourself to stop comparing yourself to others. Being conscious of your strengths gives you more confidence, allowing you to focus on soul healing.

- **Make Yourself Your Biggest Competitor**

    It is all too tempting to judge yourself against others or to wonder if you are as productive as they are. When in truth, setting up a competition between yourself is the best method to drive yourself to do more. Consider your current situation and the objectives you have set for yourself: how can you get from here to there?

    Keep a notebook because it helps you to collect your thoughts. Journaling is one of the best techniques to quit comparing yourself to others. You learn to focus on what you have accomplished rather than what others have accomplished, and you only compete with yourself as a result. This type of healthy competition allows you to be more at ease with yourself and appreciate what you have to offer.

- **Take a Social Media Break**

Nowadays, most people start making comparisons after spending a significant amount of time on social media. Though social media allows you to communicate with your loved ones, it is also beneficial to retain your distance from such platforms from time to time.

You must set boundaries the moment you realize that social media is harming your mental health in order to stop comparing yourself to others. Instead of looking through social media and making comparisons, spend an hour doing activities you enjoy each day. It will allow you to focus on doing things that make you happy rather than worrying about not being enough.

- **Give Yourself Enough Credit**

You are already doing your best, and it is past time for you to start rewarding yourself for your achievements. Rather than comparing yourself to others, be grateful for the life you have created for yourself.

Despite the fact that you are still a long way from where you want to be, you have started your self-love journey. When did you appreciate yourself the last time for everything you have accomplished thus far? Forget about what she is doing; she is not you. Tell yourself that you will achieve a lot more in the future because you will.

This type of positive thinking will help you stop comparing yourself to others and heal from all of the pain you have experienced.

There is only one of you. Take pride in your uniqueness.

Cultivate Authenticity

In this screen-obsessed culture, being your true self might feel scary. We are simply attempting to blend in, be liked, and be accepted by other people. As a result, the images we display (on our social media pages and in-person) have become merely projections of who we think we should be rather than true reflections of who we are. So, how can we remove the mask we have been wearing and begin to live a life that is true to ourselves?

- **Observe Yourself Objectively**

  According to psychology, we were sculpted as children by our parents, religions, schools, and peers to become "acceptable" in their eyes. It did not matter how that pressure twisted us. The use of social media has exacerbated this trend. We developed our system of beliefs as a result of all of this learning and pressure, and the "Adaptive Self" was born.

  To restore your "Authentic Self," you must observe how your "Adaptive Self" behaves, what it believes, how it behaves under pressure, and how it responds to obstacles as you live your life in the present. Suppose you want to make any changes at the deepest level of your being. In that case, you must first rethink your beliefs, values and behavior. You will find out if your actions and attitudes are simply the strategies you adopted years ago to fit in better or actually improving your life. By recognizing adaptive coping behaviors like defensiveness, seeking attention, or trying to satisfy others, you will start to recognize the falsehood and discover the glimmers of truth behind it.

- **Examine False Beliefs**

You were easily molded when you were younger, but now that you are an adult exploring your own inner terrain, you will quickly notice inconsistencies in your beliefs. You can let go of the false belief if you acknowledge what is true for you right now. That is living your life according to the needs of your inner self rather than the dictates of society or the programming you received as a youngster.

- **Open Conversation Between the Adaptive and Authentic Self**

Here's one to try if you enjoy visualization exercises. Use your imagination to invite two sides of your psyche - the "Authentic Self" and the "Adaptive Self" - for an inner mind discussion, whether you want to see, hear or feel. Respectfully introduce both: express gratitude to the "Adaptive Self" for assisting you in navigating some difficult and perplexing situations. Please note that there are no negative implications here.

Invite the "Authentic Self" to come forward now. Once you have developed a clearer understanding of how you may have "lost your way" in a sea of beliefs, apologize for not being truly true to yourself in the past and commit to doing better. Are you willing to listen to both sides if you truly want to improve your personal authenticity? Invite both parties to join in this debate in your mind's eye. Mentally ask a question while encouraging each side to express themselves fully and then attentively listen to the responses. Encourage discussion so that you can understand both sides of the argument. This may help you understand why you believe what you believe and which ones you no longer believe and are ready to discard.

- **Develop Effective Communication**

Improving your communication skills can help you live a more honest life.

What we want to communicate is frequently overshadowed by how we say it. According to Judith E. Glaser's research, nine out of ten discussions are ineffective. Miscommunication, conflicts, and uncertainties occur when the other person does not grasp our intentions.

Some people are passive communicators who keep their ideas to themselves. Others try to take over conversations and do not listen. Sarcasm and dishonesty are barriers to genuine communication among passive-aggressive communicators.

- **Take a Break to Understand Better**

  It makes sense to use all of your mental resources to discover a solution when you are stuck. However, such a technique can sometimes lead to nowhere and a cycle of overthinking. Taking a break allows you to listen to your heart and gut instincts, and answers will come to you naturally.

Are you sure you want to spend your whole life living up to others' standards and wishes when it is actually YOUR life?

Live in the Moment

Every day, our minds jump from what we are doing right now to our phone ringing, something that happened yesterday, someone walking into our office, and so on.

All of this mental bouncing is taxing, especially considering that the bulk of our thoughts is negative. According to some estimates, we have roughly 45,000 negative ideas per day, accounting for 80 percent of all our thoughts. Consider how this affects your emotions, as well as your physical well-being. So here are some tips for you:

- **Observe Your Surroundings**

  Observing your environment is one approach to being in the present moment. How frequently do you stop what you are doing to look around and observe what's going on? Take advantage of this moment by closing both eyes and taking a deep breath, then opening them and taking in your surroundings.

> - What do you think about the walls?

> - What about the floor or ceiling — can you find any patterns there?

> - To your left and right, how many windows do you have?

> - How many lights can you count?

It is easier to live in the present moment when you take a moment to glance around and take in everything around you.

- **Be Grateful for What You Have**

Being grateful for what you have today is an important part of living in the present moment.

If you are always thinking about what you do not have, you are not taking the time to appreciate what you do have right now.

Writing a list of things you are grateful for and reviewing it on a daily basis is one approach to practicing gratitude. Make a list of at least three things you are grateful for in your life. You may also go on a thankfulness binge, where you write down as many things as you can think of in a set amount of time.

- **Do not Multitask**

While multitasking and working on numerous activities at once may appear to be more productive, constantly juggling multiple projects makes it difficult to live in the present moment. While completing something that takes your undivided attention may appear daunting at first, be mindful of how your productivity increases when you are completely focused on a task. Consider trying to cram a lot of things into a short period of time or devoting half of your efforts to three different projects.

Put your full focus on whatever you are working on. According to studies, when you are completely concentrated on what is going on at the time, you can remember things better in the long run.

- **Let Go of Expectations**

If you want to begin living in the present moment, you must let go of your expectations and accept things as they are. You cannot control and regulate everything that happens around you; life will sometimes turn out differently than you expected. Acceptance practice will assist you in letting go of things in your life that are beyond your control.

- **Mindfulness Meditation**

Developing a daily meditation practice can make you more aware of your feelings and thoughts, allowing you to spend more time in the present moment.

You should be aware of everything you do, from eating to looking through your phone. Instead, try to concentrate on each meal while you eat it.

> ➤ What is the smell of the food?

> What does it taste like?

> What are the sounds around you when you eat - phone calls, outside traffic noises, music playing in the background?

> What is your body's reaction to the food you have eaten thus far?

- **Make Positive Company**

Surrounding oneself with positive, encouraging people will boost your own happiness and positivity. As a result, instead of obsessing on past or future events, you will be able to concentrate on what is going well right now.

Please understand that you have no control over your past, and you can only have the future you dream of by living in the present. Ultimately, the present is all you have, and it needs your most attention.

You can show yourself the love and acceptance you need by following these strategies.

Conclusion

"Imagine two carriages, each marked with a couple of short words: 'Self-Esteem' on one, and 'Self-Confidence' on the other, similar to my child's train set. These carriages are constantly circling the little circular track, with no clear way to change direction. They cannot move somewhere new; in fact, they're stuck in the same loop over and over again. And this is something that genuinely frightens me." This is how a young mother recently explained her feelings to me. It was poetic and heartfelt.

It is sad that women often have a lot of self-limiting ideas that keep them from taking the required steps toward personal fulfillment and pleasure. Girls frequently have lower self-esteem, lesser life expectations, and less confidence in their talents and in themselves than boys when they reach adolescence.

You can develop confidence in yourself as a woman to push yourself further in your abilities. The first and most critical ingredient in the personal change formula is taking personal responsibility for changing your negative thoughts. Only you have the power to bring new and exciting experiences into your life. It is a task, and you will need to persist with it if you want to succeed.

Change that lasts and is significant does not occur as a result of every action you take in life. A single failed attempt would set you back a long way if this were the case. True self-esteem and self-confidence come from knowing that you are in charge and that you can fully trust yourself to take action and see it through, no matter what happens.

"Her Motivational Code" is focused on giving women a helping hand in aligning their confidence to their potential in every field of life.

The first chapter of this book deals with women and self-doubt. It discusses what issues might be hiding behind your self-doubt as imposter syndrome, self-sabotaging, a lack of compassion, etc. It further includes strategies to overcome your self-doubt, e.g., identifying and replacing limiting beliefs, saying "No" to being powerless, cultivating self-compassion, letting go of perfectionism, working on self-awareness, finding validation from within, and avoiding self-criticism, etc.

The second chapter is devoted to boosting confidence in women. It includes reasons why self-confidence matters and then moves on to effective ways to achieve it: finding out what confidence feels like, finding the root cause, designing your ideal life, learning to love your body, adopting a growth mindset, and photo-shopping your self-image and boosting competency, etc.

The third chapter is about self-acceptance and self-love. The first section explains the absurd standard of "perfect" as fiction. The second section includes strategies to embrace yourself, such as practicing true self-love, redefining happiness, avoiding comparison, cultivating authenticity, and living in the moment.

I have put together this book with love which I hope reflects on you. If you have found this book helpful in your journey towards self-love and self-acceptance, please leave a review on Amazon.